THE MODERN MEDITERRANEAN COOKBOOK

A Diet That Combines the Seasonability, Locality, and Good Taste of Aliments Into Delicious Dishes!

Mediterranean Flavor

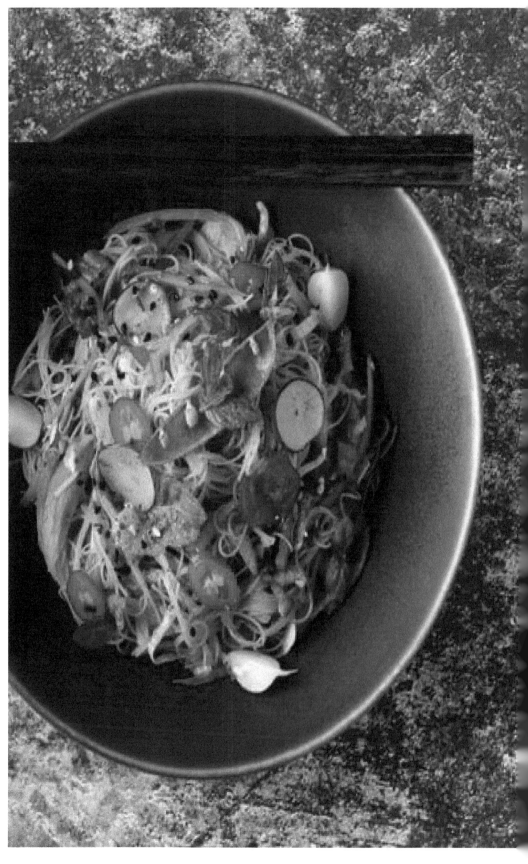

Table of Contents

INTRODUCTION

The Mediterranean Diet is the traditional diet of the countries surrounding the Mediterranean Sea, such as Greece, Spain, and Italy. It focuses on the regional foods from those countries, which have many benefits, including improving heart health, chronic disease, and obesity.

The Mediterranean Diet reflects the personality of these regions and includes a wonderful variety of ingredients and recipes, featuring grains, fats from fish, olive oil, nuts, fruits, and lean meats. It is easy to follow and will provide lots of healthy and delicious meals that your family will love.

This diet is generally characterized by a high intake of plant-based food such as fresh fruits, vegetables, nuts and cereals, and olive oil, with a moderate amount of fish and poultry, and a small amount of dairy products, red meats, and sweets. Wine is allowed with every meal but at a moderate level. The Mediterranean Diet focuses strongly on social and cultural activities like communal mealtimes, resting after eating, and physical activities.

The Mediterranean Diet is not simply a weight loss or fad diet; however, raising your dietary fiber and cutting down on red meat, animal fats, and processed foods will lead to weight loss and a decreased risk of many diseases.

The Mediterranean Diet Pyramid

The Mediterranean Diet Pyramid is a visual tool that summarizes the diet. It suggests pattern of eating and gives guidelines for meal frequency and food management. This pyramid allows you to develop healthy eating habits and maintain calorie counts as well.

The pyramid tiers consist of the following groups:

- **Plant-based foods**

This includes olive oil, fruits, vegetables, whole grains, legumes, beans, nuts and seeds, and spices and herbs. These foods should be part of every meal. Olive oil is the main fat used in cooking. It can occasionally be replaced with butter or cooking oil, but in smaller quantities.

Fresh herbs and spices can be used in generous amounts in dishes for enhancing taste and as an alternative to salt. Dried herbs can also be used. Fresh ginger and garlic are always allowed for flavor.

- **Seafood**

Seafood is an important staple and one of the main sources of protein in the Mediterranean Diet. Make sure you have seafood at least twice a week. There are many varieties of fish that will work, as well as mussels, shrimps, and crab. Tuna is a great source of protein and works well in sandwiches and salads.

- **Dairy and Poultry**

Yogurt, milk, cheese, and poultry can be consumed ata moderate level. If you use eggs in cooking and baking, include them in your weekly limit. Choose healthy cheese options like ricotta, feta, and Parmesan. You can have them as toppings and garnishing your meals and dishes.

- **Sweets and Red Meat**

Sweets and meats are used less in this diet. If you eat them, cut down on the quantity and choose lean meat. Red meat, sugar, and fat are not good for heart health and blood sugar.

- **Water**

The Mediterranean Diet encourages increased daily water intake, 9 8-ounce glasses for women and 13 for men. For pregnant and breastfeeding women, the amount should be higher.

- **Wine**

The Mediterranean Diet allows for moderate wine consumption with meals. Alcohol reduces the risk of heart disease. One glass of wine for women and two for men is the recommended daily limit.

Foods That Are Not Allowed in the Mediterranean Diet

This diet satisfies your food cravings by providing better alternatives. It helps you to shift your mindset from looking for snacks to having fresh fruits and vegetables that will satisfy your between-meal hunger.

The following items should be restricted or replaced by healthy options:

- **Added sugar**

Sugar is one of the most difficult items to avoid in your diet. Try to stick to healthy sugar from fresh fruits and vegetables. Avoid processed foods; the added sugars in pasta sauce, peanut butter, fruit juices, bread, and bakery products are considered empty calories.

Added sugars are commonly used in processed food like:

- High fructose corn syrup
- Glucose
- Corn syrup

- Sucrose
- Maltose
- Corn sweetener

You can add fresh fruits like strawberries and raspberries to your water for flavor and refreshment as well as eating them. Switch to an organic sweetener like honey or maple syrup instead of using refined sugars.

- **Refined grains**

Refined grains are prohibited in the Mediterranean Diet because they lead to heart disease and type 2 diabetes. Grains are often grouped with carbohydrates, but they do not fall into the "bad carbs" category until they are refined. Refined grains go through a milling process during which the major nutrients are removed. They are left with less fiber, iron, and vitamins and more empty calories.

The most common refined grains consist of:

- White flour
- White bread
- White rice
- White flour pizza crust

- **Breakfast cereals**

Whole grains are a better alternative. When possible, choose sourdough bread. Enjoy sandwiches in a whole-grain wrap or pita bread. You can also try plant-based alternatives like cauliflower crust, cauliflower rice, or spiralized vegetables in place of pasta. Swap in whole grains like quinoa and brown rice.

- **Refined Oils**

Refined oils are extremely damaging to your health. The key nutrients have been stripped from out and additional chemicals added in, making their way to your food.

Most oils are extracted from the seeds of plants. This includes soybean oil, corn oil, sunflower oil, peanut oil, and olive oil. Vegetable oils are a combination of multiple plants. The process of extracting the oil involves a variety of chemicals that can increase inflammation in the body. The fat that remains in the oil has been linked to several health conditions such as cancer, heart disease, and diabetes. Oils are also used to create margarine in a hydrogenation process, using chemicals that allow the oil to remain in a solid-state. When the oil is hydrogenated, the fatty acids that were in the oil are further destroyed and transformed into trans fatty acids. Several scientific studies have been conducted to show the connection of trans fatty acids to some debilitating health conditions.

Trans fatty acids are considered to be some of the unhealthiest fats you can consume, especially when it comes to your heart. These industrially manufactured fats cause LDL cholesterol to increase. High amounts of LDL or bad cholesterol can clog and destroy your arteries and increase blood pressure. This significantly increases your risk of heart attack and stroke.

Some of the most common trans fats or hydrogenated oils that you might not be aware of include:

- Microwaveable popcorn
- Butter
- Margarine
- Vegetable oil
- Fried foods
- Pre-packaged muffins, cakes, doughnuts, and pastries
- Coffee creamers
- Prepared pizza dough or pizza crust
- Cake frosting
- Potato chips
- Crackers

The Mediterranean Diet focuses on replacing these refined oils and processed foods with more wholesome and natural ingredients. Refined oils can be easy to eliminate from your diet. If you are used to sautéing your foods with refined oil, switch to unrefined olive oil. Instead of frying foods in oil, bake or grill them.

- **Processed Meat**

Processed meats have been processed extensively to preserve flavors and provide a longer shelf life. The most common forms are bacon, hot dogs, deli meats, sausage, and canned meats. Consuming processed meat daily can cause or increase the risk of colorectal cancer, stomach cancer, pancreatic cancer, and prostate cancer.

Sodium is what makes processed meats so harmful. Sodium is well known to increase blood pressure, which increases the risk of different heart diseases. Processed meat contains at least 50 percent more preservatives than unprocessed meats. These preservatives affect sugar tolerances and can cause insulin resistance, which can lead to diabetes.

- Switch out processed meats and red meats for fish or poultry.
- Use vegetables or beans in place of meat.

- Use a variety of spices to add more flavor to a dish where you would use meat in the same way.
- Spices like cumin, coriander, peppercorn, and marjoram add unique flavors to the dish so you won't miss the bacon, sausage, or ground meat.
- You can use different seasonings on sautéed or baked vegetables.
- Add roasted chickpeas or toasted seeds and nuts to dishes for more texture. These can be great alternatives to dishes that call for bacon crumbles.

Common Mistakes in the Mediterranean Diet:

When you start a new diet, you will make some mistakes or encounter situations in which you don't know what to do. Before you get on the Mediterranean Diet plan, here is a heads-up about common mistakes that people make. If you know about these mistakes, you can avoid them and achieve success more quickly.

- **All or Nothing**

Your attitude toward your diet matters a lot. This is why you must make sure you are mentally prepared for it. It will be different from your ordinary lifestyle, which is why you need an abundance of information. To learn the benefits of this diet, you can ask the experts or people who have experienced it.

- **Eating the Same Things**

Don't eat the same things over and over again, day after day. One of the most common mistakes people make is that they think that eating the same kind of vegetables all week long will help them lose weight. You must have variety in your diet. The Mediterranean Diet allows you to have multiple kinds of dishes throughout the week, but maintain portion control.

- **Deprivation**

Another mistake people make is thinking that deprivation is the only way to lose weight. The main point of this diet plan is to give you energy while helping you lose weight. Deprivation will only make you weaker. This diet plan won't work if you don't eat at all, so be sure to keep this in mind.

- **Giving up**

Don't give up in the middle of the Mediterranean Diet. If you see yourself losing weight and you think, *now I can cheat a little* … resist. Since you've put so much effort into it already, don't give up now. If you have chocolate cravings, find a healthy alternative. It's easier to develop self-control if you can see the results, so keep your goals in mind and stay strong. Our bodies need time to adjust and stabilize in terms of the food we eat, so switching back and forth is never a good option.

- **Not setting goals**

One of the main mistakes people make is not setting goals when they start the diet. You must have a goal in terms of how much weight you want to lose and work toward it. When you don't have a plan, you will become distracted and be unable to reach your destination, no matter how hard you try.

- **Following the wrong plan**

Another common mistake is that you don't have enough knowledge about the plan you are following to lose weight. Maybe you are following the wrong plan, one that doesn't seem to work for you. If you're confused, don't decide by yourself to follow the Mediterranean Diet; consult an expert who can advise you on what to eat and do to adopt a healthy lifestyle. Many people try to keep their old habits while mixing in elements of the Mediterranean Diet, but if you don't follow the diet, you won't achieve the optimal results. Decide if you're willing to do it, and then do it right.

Your Mediterranean Shopping Guide

Apart from knowing how to start your diet, it is necessary to know a little about how to set-up your food charts.

What to have:

- Fresh vegetables: tomatoes, kale, spinach, cauliflower, Brussels sprouts, cucumbers, etc.
- Fresh fruits: An orange, apples, pears, grapes, dates, strawberries, figs, peaches, etc.
- Seeds and nuts: almonds, walnuts, cashews, sunflower seeds, etc.
- Legumes: beans, lentils, chickpeas, etc.
- Roots: yams, turnips, sweet potatoes, etc.
- Whole grains: whole oats, rye, brown rice, corn, barley, buckwheat, whole wheat, whole grain pasta, and bread
- Fish and seafood: sardines, salmon, tuna, shrimp, mackerel, oyster, crab, clams, mussels, etc.
- Poultry: turkey, chicken, duck, etc.
- Eggs—chicken, duck, quail
- Dairy products such as cheese, Greek yogurt, etc.

- Herbs and spices: mint, basil, garlic, rosemary, cinnamon, sage, pepper, etc.
- Healthy fats and oil: extra virgin olive oil, avocado oil, olives, etc.

What to avoid:

- Foods with added sugar like soda, ice cream, candy, table sugar, etc.
- Refined grains like white bread or pasta made with refined wheat
- Margarine and similar processed foods that contain trans fats
- Refined oil such as cottonseed oil, soybean oil, etc.
- Processed meat such as hot dogs, sausages, bacon, etc.
- Highly processed food with labels such as "Low-Fat" or "Diet," or anything that is not natural

Useful Information about Healthy Foods

1. **Oils**

The Mediterranean Diet emphasizes healthy oils. The following are some of the oils that you might want to consider.

- **Coconut oil:** Coconut oil is semi-solid at room temperature and can be used for months without turning sour. Coconut oil also has a lot of health benefits as lauric acid, which can help to improve cholesterol levels and kill various pathogens.

- **Extra-virgin olive oil:** Olive oil is well-known worldwide as one of the healthiest oils, and it is a key ingredient in the Mediterranean Diet. Olive oil can help to improve health biomarkers such as increasing HDL cholesterol and lowering the amount of bad LDL cholesterol.

- **Avocado oil:** Avocado oil is very similar to olive oil and has similar health benefits. It can be used for many purposes as an alternative to olive oil (such as in cooking).

2. Healthy salt alternatives and spices

Aside from replacing healthy oils, the Mediterranean Diet will allow you to opt for healthy salt alternatives as well.

- **Sunflower seeds**

Sunflower seeds are excellent and give a nutty and sweet flavor.

- **Fresh squeezed lemon**

Lemon is packed with Vitamin C, which helps to neutralize damaging free radicals from the system.

- **Onion powder**

Onion powder is a dehydrated ground spice made from an onion bulb, which is mostly used as a seasoning and is a fine salt alternative.

- **Black pepper**

Black pepper is also a salt alternative that is native to India. It is made by grinding whole peppercorns.

- **Cinnamon**

Cinnamon is well-known as a savory spice and available in two varieties: Ceylon and Chinese. Both of them sport a sharp, warm, and sweet flavor.

- **Fruit-infused vinegar**

Fruit-infused vinegar or flavored vinegar can give a nice flavor to meals. These are excellent ingredients to add a bit of flavor to meals without salt.

Eating Out on the Mediterranean Diet

It might seem a bit confusing, but eating out at a restaurant while on a Mediterranean Diet is pretty easy. Just follow the simple rules below:

- Try to ensure that you choose seafood or fish as the main dish of your meal
- When ordering, try to make a special request and ask the restaurant to fry their food using extra virgin olive oil
- Ask for only whole-grain based ingredients if possible
- If possible, try to read the menu before going to the restaurant
- Try to have a simple snack before you go out; this will help prevent you from overeating.

BREAKFAST

Stewed Eggplant

2 Servings

Preparation Time: 35 Minutes

Ingredients:

- 6 tbsps extra-virgin olive oil
- 1 medium white onion, chopped
- 4 large carrots, sliced diagonally
- 8 medium Italian eggplant, trimmed
- 4 large potatoes, peeled and diced
- 1 large tomato, diced
- 1 (16-oz.) can tomato sauce
- 1 tsp. garlic powder
- 1 tsp. paprika
- 1½ tsps of salt
- 2 cups fresh cilantro, chopped

Directions:

- In a 3-quart pot over medium heat, heat extra-virgin olive oil. Add white onion and carrots, and cook for 5 minutes.
- Add Italian eggplant and potatoes, and cook for 7 minutes.
- Add tomato, and cook for 3 minutes.

- Add tomato sauce, garlic powder, paprika, and salt, and simmer, stirring occasionally, for 15 minutes.
- Stir in cilantro, and cook for 5 more minutes.
- Serve with brown rice.

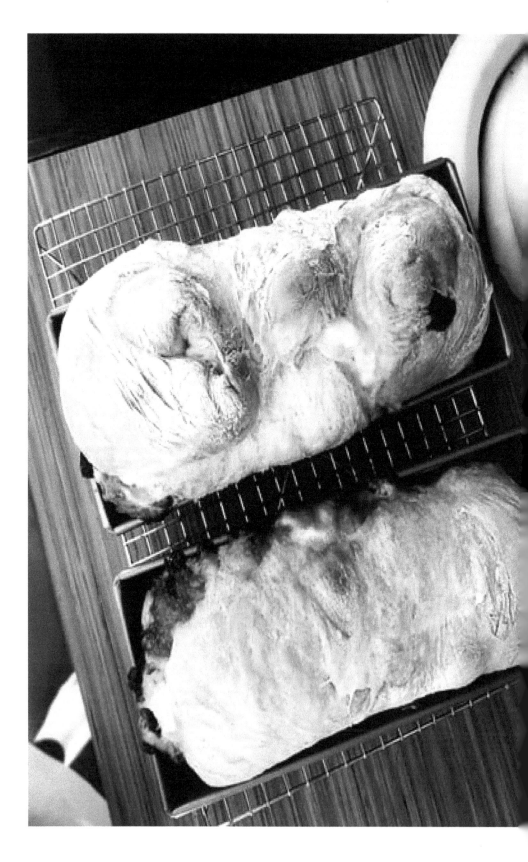

Valentine's Pancakes

4 Servings

Preparation Time: 20 Minutes

Ingredients:
- 8 eggs, preferably organic
- 4 pieces banana, peeled and then cut into small pieces
- 1 teaspoon extra-virgin olive oil (for the pancake pan)
- 1 tablespoon milled flax seeds, preferably organic
- 1 tablespoon bee pollen, milled, preferably organic

Directions:
- Crack the eggs into a mixing bowl. Add in the banana, flax seeds, and bee pollen. With a hand mixer, blend the ingredients until smooth batter inn texture.
- Put a few drops of the olive oil in a nonstick pancake pan over medium flame or heat. Pour some batter into the pan; cook for about 2 minutes, undisturbed until the bottom of the pancake is golden and can be lifted easily from the pan. With a silicon spatula, lift and flip the

pancake; cook for about 30seconds more and transfer into a plate.

- Repeat the process with the remaining batter, oiling the pan with every new batter.
- Serve the pancake as you cook or serve them all together topped with vanilla, strawberry, pine nuts jam.

Chocolate Banana Bread

20 Servings

Preparation Time: 50 Minutes

Ingredients:

- ¼ cup dark chocolate, chopped
- 1 cup almond butter
- 1 cup coconut flour, sifted
- ½ teaspoon cinnamon powder
- 2 teaspoons baking soda
- 1 teaspoon vanilla extract
- 8 bananas, mashed
- 8 eggs
- 8 tablespoons coconut oil, melted
- A pinch of salt

Directions:

- Preheat the oven to 350oF.
- Grease an 8" x 8" square pan and set aside.
- In a large bowl, mix together the eggs, banana, vanilla extract, almond butter and coconut oil. Mix well until well combined.
- Add the cinnamon powder, coconut flour, baking powder, baking soda and salt to the wet ingredients. Fold until well combined. Add in the chopped chocolates then fold the batter again.

- Pour the batter into the greased pan. Spread evenly.
- Bake in the oven for about 50 minutes or until a toothpick inserted in the center comes out clean.
- Remove from the hot oven and cool in a wire rack for an hour.

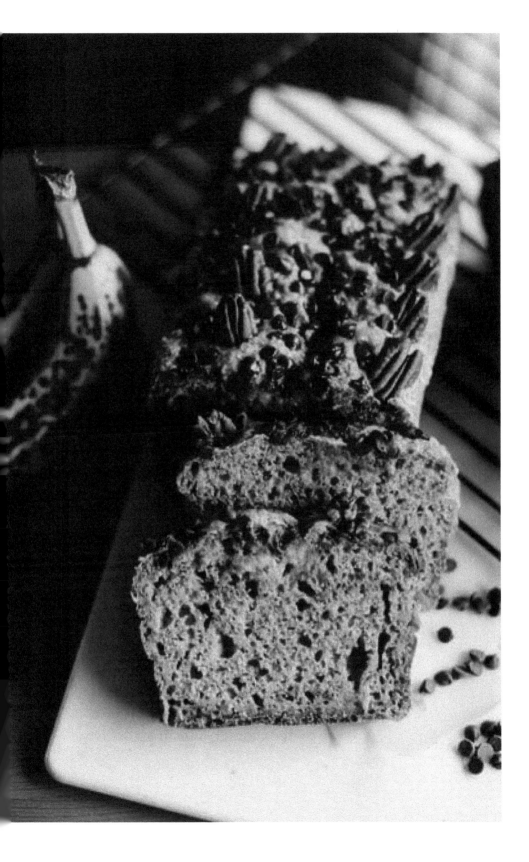

Fresh Greek Yogurt

2 Servings

Preparation Time: 20 Minutes

Ingredients:

- 2 gal whole milk
- 4 cups plain Greek yogurt

Directions:

- In a large pot over medium-low heat, bring whole milk to a simmer until a froth starts to form on the surface. If you have a thermometer, bring the milk to 185ºF.
- Remove from heat, and let the milk cool to lukewarm, or 110ºF.
- Pour all but about 2 cups of milk into a large plastic container.
- Pour the remaining 2 cups of milk into a smaller bowl. Add Greek yogurt, and stir until well combined.
- Slowly pour milk and yogurt mixture into the large bowl of milk, and stir well.
- Cover the bowl with a lid, and set it aside where it won't be disturbed. Cover it with a towel, and let it sit overnight.
- The next morning, gently transfer the bowl to the refrigerator. Chill for at least 1 day.

- The next day, gently pour off clear liquid that's formed on top of yogurt, leaving just a little liquid remaining.
- Serve, or store in the refrigerator for up to 2 weeks.

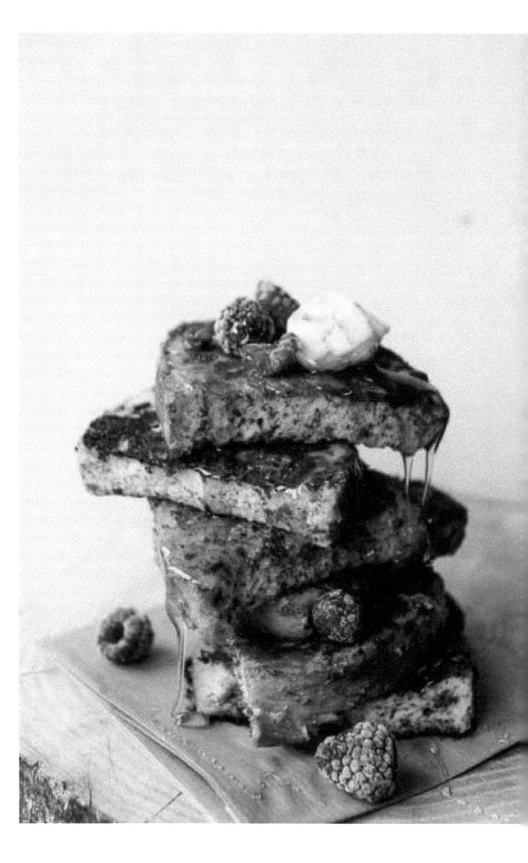

Eggs with Pepper, Dill, and Salmon

12 Servings

Preparation Time: 15 Minutes

Ingredients:

- Pepper and salt to taste
- 2 tsps red pepper flakes
- 4 garlic cloves, minced
- 1 cup crumbled goat cheese
- 2 tbsps fresh chives, chopped
- 2 tbsps fresh dill, chopped
- 4 tomatoes, diced
- 16 eggs, whisked
- 1 tsp coconut oil

Directions:

- In a big bowl, whisk the eggs. Mix in pepper, salt, red pepper flakes, garlic, dill, and salmon.
- On low fire, place a nonstick fry pan and lightly grease with oil.
- Pour egg mixture and whisk around until cooked through to make scrambled eggs.
- Serve and enjoy topped with goat cheese.

Spinach and Avocado Breakfast Wrap

8 Servings

Preparation Time: 10 Minutes

Ingredients:

- ¼ tsp pepper
- 1 tsp salt
- 2 oz box or bag of baby spinach, chopped
- 1 avocado, sliced
- 8 eggs whites
- 8 eggs
- 4 oz shredded pepper jack cheese
- 8 thin, whole wheat pita bread, 8-inch
- Hot sauce, optional
- Nonstick cooking spray

Directions:

- On medium-high fire, place a nonstick skillet greased with cooking spray.
- Once hot, sauté spinach for 2 minutes or until wilted.
- Meanwhile, in a small bowl, whisk egg whites and eggs. Season with pepper and salt, whisk again. Pour into skillet and scramble. Cook for 3 to 4 minutes or to desired doneness.

- Evenly divide egg into 4 equal portions and place in the middle of pita bread and add 2 to 4 slices of avocadoes beside the egg and roll tortilla like a burrito.
- Serve and enjoy with a side of hot sauce.

Red Pepper and Kale Frittata

8 Servings

Preparation Time: 23 Minutes

Ingredients:

- Salt and pepper to taste
- ½ cup almond milk
- 16 large eggs
- 3 cups kale, rinsed and chopped
- 6 slices of crispy bacon, chopped
- 1 cup onion, chopped
- ½ cup red pepper, chopped
- 1 tablespoon coconut oil

Directions:

- Preheat the oven to 350F.
- In a medium bowl, combine the eggs and almond milk. Season with salt and pepper. Set aside.
- In a skillet, heat the coconut oil over medium flame and sauté the onions and red pepper for three minutes or until the onion is translucent. Add in the kale and cook for 5 minutes more.

- Add the eggs into the mixture along with the bacon and cook for four minutes or until the edges start to set.
- Continue cooking the frittata in the oven for 15 minutes.

Bacon with Beans

6 Servings

Preparation Time: 30 Minutes

Ingredients:

- 6 medium sausages
- 6 bacon slices
- 4 eggs
- 2 cans baked beans
- 6 bread slices, toasted

Directions:

- Preheat the Airfryer at 325 degrees F and place sausages and bacon in a fryer basket.
- Cook for about 10 minutes and place the baked beans in a ramekin.
- Place eggs in another ramekin and the Airfryer to 395 degrees F.
- Cook for about 10 more minutes and divide the sausage mixture, beans, and eggs on serving plates
- Serve with bread slices.

LUNCH

36

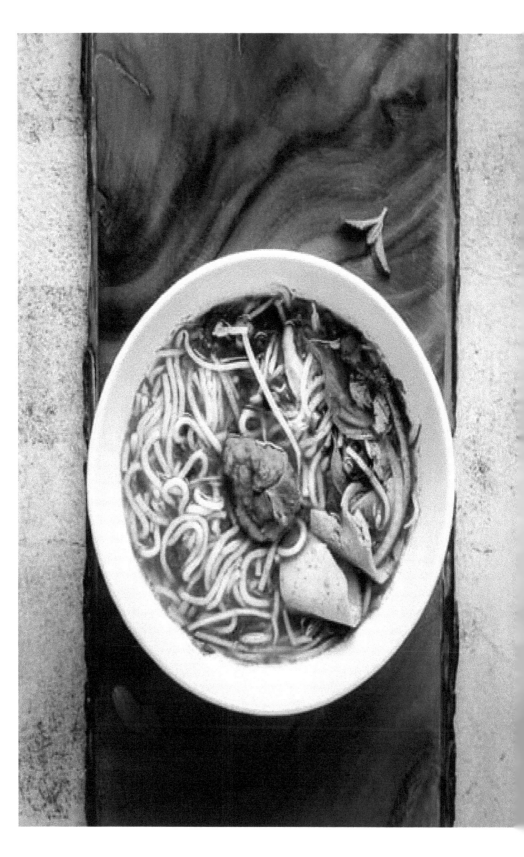

10 Servings

Preparation Time: 5 Minutes

Ingredients:

- 2 cans (25 ounces) chickpeas, drained and then rinsed
- 2 garlic cloves
- 6 tablespoons tahini
- 6 tablespoons olive oil
- 2 tablespoons lemon juice
- 1 teaspoon salt

Directions:

- Put all the ingredients in a food processor or a blender; process or blend until the texture is pasty.

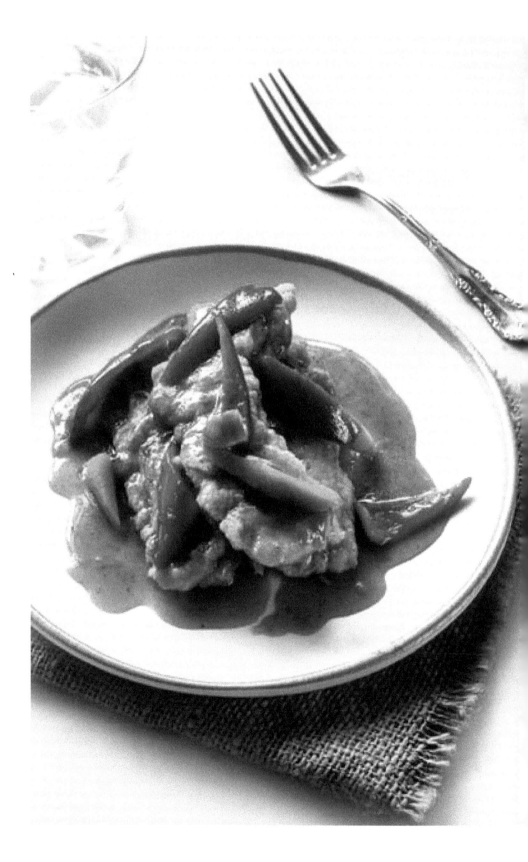

Mediterranean Vegetables

16 Servings

Preparation Time: 25 Minutes

Ingredients:

- 12 zucchini and/or yellow squash sliced into 1 inch thick (about 2 1/2 pounds total),
- 4 cups couscous
- 4 bunches scallions, trimmed
- 1 cup olive oil
- 1 quart cherry tomatoes (preferably on the vine)
- 1 large eggplant, sliced into 1/4-inch thick (about 1 pound)
- Kosher salt and black pepper
- Spiced Chili Oil or store-bought harissa (North African chili sauce, found in the international aisle)

Directions:

- Cook the couscous according to the directions on the package.
- Meanwhile, preheat the grill to medium.
- In a large-sized bowl, toss the squash, zucchini, tomatoes, eggplant, and scallions with 1 teaspoon of salt, 1/2 teaspoon of pepper, and olive oil.

- Working in batches, grill the veggies, covered, occasionally turning, until tender. The squash and the eggplant will be done after about 4-6 minutes. The scallions and the tomatoes will be done after about 1-2 minutes.
- Serve with the couscous and drizzle with the spiced chili oil.

Grilled Chicken with Oregano

8 Servings

Preparation Time: 15 Minutes

Ingredients:

- 8 boneless skinless chicken breast halves
- 3 tablespoons lemon juice
- 6 tablespoons olive oil
- 3 tablespoons chopped fresh parsley
- 6 garlic cloves, crushed and minced
- 1 teaspoon paprika
- 1 teaspoon dried oregano
- 1 teaspoon salt
- 1 teaspoon pepper

Directions:

- In a large Ziplock bag, mix well oregano, paprika, garlic, parsley, olive oil, and lemon juice.
- Pierce chicken with knife several times and sprinkle with salt and pepper.
- Add chicken to bag and marinate 20 minutes or up to two days in the fridge.
- Remove chicken from bag and grill for 5 minutes per side in a 350oF preheated grill.
- Remove chicken from grill and let it stand on a plate for 5 minutes before slicing.
- Serve and enjoy with a side of rice or salad.

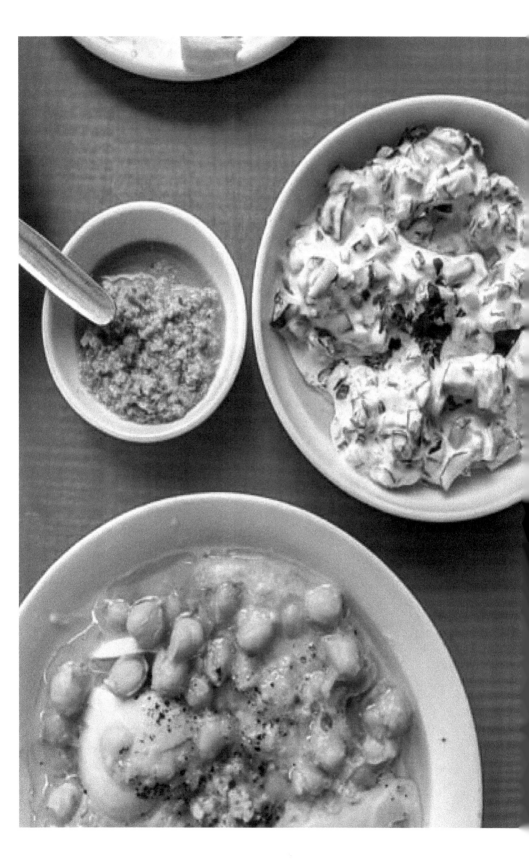

Grilled Chicken and Veggies

6 Servings

Preparation Time: 20 Minutes

Ingredients:

- ¼ teaspoon cayenne pepper
- 1 teaspoon garlic granules
- ½ teaspoon onion powder
- 2 cups organic tomatoes, blended
- 1 red onion
- 1 red pepper, chopped
- 1 tablespoon vinegar
- 2 teaspoons Italian seasoning
- 1 teaspoon rosemary
- 1 yellow squash, chopped
- 1 zucchini, chopped
- 1-pound organic chicken breast
- 4 cups fresh cherry tomatoes, halved
- 8 tablespoons extra-virgin olive oil
- Pepper to taste
- Salt to taste

Directions:

- Marinade the chicken by mixing together 1 tablespoon of extra virgin olive oil, Italian seasoning, and rosemary. Season with salt, then set aside for at least 2 hours.

- In another bowl, make the salad by combining the red onion, fresh cherry tomatoes, red pepper, squash, and zucchini. Add 1 tablespoon of extra virgin olive oil and season with salt and pepper to taste. Place inside a greased tinfoil, then set aside.
- Prepare the grill and heat it to 350F. Cook the chicken breast and let it cook for 7 minutes on each side. Place the tinfoil with the veggies on the grill and cook it for five to 7 minutes.
- Meanwhile, make the vinaigrette by combining the cayenne pepper, onion powder, garlic granules, vinegar, and blended organic tomatoes in a food processor. Add 2 tablespoons of extra virgin olive oil and season with salt and pepper to taste.

Lamb Artichokes

12 Servings

Preparation Time: 8 Hours and 5 Minutes

Ingredients:
- 4 pounds lamb shoulder, boneless and roughly cubed
- 2 spring onions, chopped
- 1 tablespoon olive oil
- 6 garlic cloves, minced
- 1 tablespoon lemon juice
- Salt and black pepper to the taste
- 1 and ½ cups veggie stock
- 12 ounces canned artichoke hearts, drained and quartered
- 1 cup feta cheese, crumbled
- 2 tablespoons parsley, chopped

Directions:
- Heat up a pan with the oil over medium-high heat, add the lamb, brown 5 minutes, and transfer to your slow cooker.
- Add the rest of the ingredients except the parsley and the cheese, put the lid on, and cook on Low for 8 hours.
- Add the cheese and the parsley, divide the mix between plates and serve.

Mix Lamb and Plums

8 Servings

Preparation Time: 6 Hours and 10 Minutes

Ingredients:

- 8 lamb shanks
- 1 red onion, chopped
- 4 tablespoons olive oil
- 1 cup plum, pitted and halved
- 1 tablespoon sweet paprika
- 4 cups chicken stock
- Salt and pepper to the taste

Directions:

- Heat up a pan with the oil over medium-high heat, add the lamb, brown for 5 minutes on each side, and transfer to your slow cooker.
- Add the rest of the ingredients, put the lid on, and cook on high heat for 6 hours.
- Divide the mix between plates and serve right away.

Lamb with Mango Sauce

8 Servings

Preparation Time: 1 Hour

Ingredients:
- 4 cups Greek yogurt
- 1 cup mango, peeled and cubed
- 2 yellow onions, chopped
- 1 cup parsley, chopped
- 1 pound lamb, cubed
- ½ teaspoon red pepper flakes
- Salt and black pepper to the taste
- 4 tablespoons olive oil
- ¼ teaspoon cinnamon powder

Directions:
- Heat up a pan with the oil over medium-high heat, add the meat, and brown for 5 minutes.
- Add the onion and sauté for 5 minutes more.
- Add the rest of the ingredients, toss, bring to a simmer and cook over medium heat for 45 minutes.
- Divide everything between plates and serve.

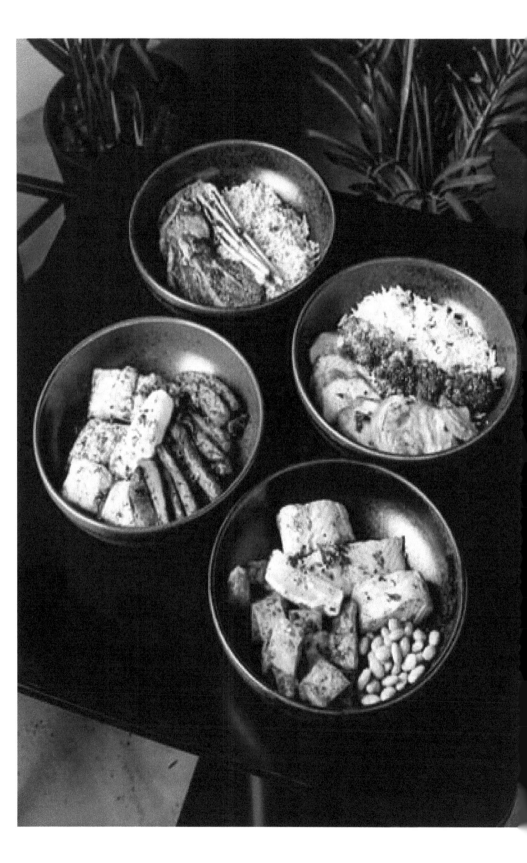

Pork Chops with Mix Cherries

8 Servings

Preparation Time: 12 Minutes

Ingredients:

- 8 pork chops, boneless
- Salt and black pepper to the taste
- 1 cup cranberry juice
- 2 and ½ teaspoons spicy mustard
- 1 cup dark cherries, pitted and halved
- Cooking spray

Directions:

- Heat up a pan greased with the cooking spray over medium-high heat, add the pork chops, cook them for 5 minutes on each side, and divide between plates.
- Heat up the same pan over medium heat, add the cranberry juice and the rest of the ingredients, whisk, bring to a simmer, cook for 2 minutes, drizzle over the pork chops and serve.

Lamb Barley Mix

8 Servings

Preparation Time: 8 Hours and 10 Minutes

Ingredients:

- 4 tablespoons olive oil
- 1 cup barley soaked overnight, drained, and rinsed
- 2 pounds lamb meat, cubed
- 1 red onion, chopped
- 8 garlic cloves, minced
- 6 carrots, chopped
- 12 tablespoons dill, chopped
- 2 tablespoons tomato paste
- 6 cups veggie stock
- A pinch of salt and black pepper

Directions:

- Heat up a pan with the oil over medium-high heat, add the meat, brown for 5 minutes on each side and transfer to your slow cooker.
- Add the barley and the rest of the ingredients, put the lid on, and cook on low heat for 8 hours.
- Divide everything between plates and serve.

BRUNCH

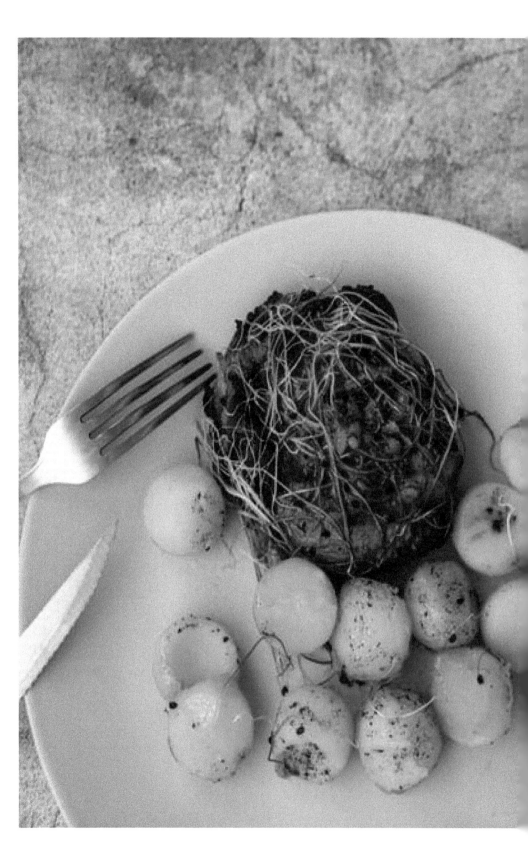

Fresh Baba Ganoush

4 Servings

Preparation Time: 50 Minutes

Ingredients:
- 4 large eggplants
- 8 tbs extra-virgin olive oil
- 1 large white onion, chopped
- 2 tbsps minced garlic
- 4 tbsps fresh lemon juice
- 1 tsp. salt
- 1 tsp ground black pepper
- 1 medium red bell pepper, ribs and seeds removed, and finely diced
- 1 medium green bell pepper, ribs, and seeds removed, and finely diced
- 3 tbsps fresh parsley, finely chopped
- 1 tsp cayenne

Directions:
- 3 medium radishes, finely diced
- 3 whole green onions, finely chopped
- Preheat a grill top or a grill to medium-low heat.
- Place eggplants on the grill, and roast on all sides for 40 minutes, turning every 5 minutes. Immediately place eggplants on a

plate, cover with plastic wrap, let cool for 15 minutes.

- Remove eggplant stems, and peel off as much skin as possible. (It's okay if it doesn't all come off.)
- In a food processor fitted with a chopping blade, pulse eggplant 7 times. Transfer eggplant to a medium bowl.
- In a medium saucepan over low heat, heat 2 tablespoons extra-virgin olive oil. Add white onion, and sauté, occasionally stirring for 10 minutes. Add onions to the eggplant.
- Add garlic, lemon juice, salt, black pepper, red bell pepper, green bell pepper, and parsley to eggplant, and stir well.
- Spread baba ganoush on a serving plate, and drizzle the remaining 2 tablespoons extra-virgin olive oil over the top. Sprinkle with cayenne, radishes, and green onions.
- Serve cold or at room temperature.

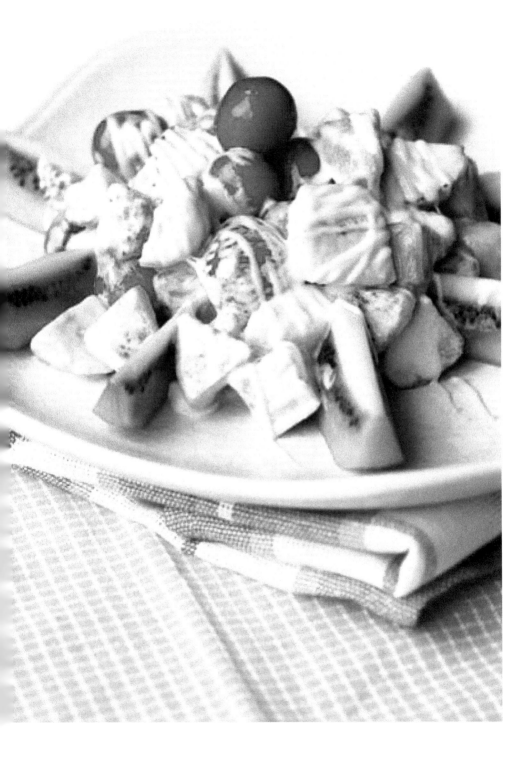

Mediterranean Chicken Tabbouleh

4 Servings

Preparation Time: 30 Minutes

Ingredients:

- 12 ounces chicken breast halves, skinless, boneless, broiled or grilled, then sliced
- 8 large leaves romaine and/or butterhead (Bibb or Boston) lettuce
- 1 cup water
- 3 tablespoons lemon juice
- 4 tablespoons olive oil
- 2 tablespoons green onions, thinly sliced
- 1/8 teaspoon ground black pepper
- 1 teaspoon salt
- 1 cup bulgur
- 1 cup tomato (1 medium), chopped
- 1 cup seeded cucumber, finely chopped
- 1 cup Italian parsley, finely chopped
- 1 tablespoon fresh mint, snipped (or 1 teaspoon dried mint, crushed)

Directions:

- In a large-sized bowl, combine the bulgur and the water; let stand for 30 minutes. After 30 minutes, drain in the sink through a fine sieve, pressing out the excess water from the bulgur using a large spoon. Return the bulgur into the bowl. Stir in the cucumber, tomatoes, green onions, parsley, and mint.

- Prepare the dressing; put the olive oil, lemon juice, salt, and pepper into a screw-top jar. Cover securely and shake well until well mixed. Pour the dressing over the bulgur mixture; lightly toss to coat the bulgur mixture with the dressing. Cover the bowl and refrigerate to chill for at least 4 hours up to 24 hours, occasionally stirring.
- When ready to serve, bring the bulgur mixture to room temperature. Divide the romaine and/or butterhead lettuce leaves between 2 shallow bowls, top with the broiled or grilled chicken, and then top with the bulgur mixture.

Tahini Silky Sauce

8 Servings

Preparation Time: 15 Minutes

Ingredients:
- 2 cups tahini sesame seed paste, made from light colored seeds
- ¼ cup freshly squeezed lemon juice, or more to taste
- ¼ teaspoon salt, or more to taste
- 6 cloves raw garlic (or 5 cloves roasted garlic)
- 1 cup lukewarm water, or more for consistency
- 4 teaspoons fresh parsley, minced, optional

Directions:
- Put the tahini paste, lemon juice, lukewarm water, and salt in the food processor; process, scraping the sides periodically until the mixture is ivory-colored and creamy.
- If using a blender, break the thick parts of the mixture every 30 seconds using a long-handled spoon; this will prevent the blender blades from clogging.
- Process or blend until the sauce turns into a smooth, rich paste.

- If the mixture is too thick, slowly add water until the texture is according to your desired consistency.
- If using tahini as a topping for a meat dish or hummus, make the sauce creamy and thick.
- If using as a condiment for falafel or fits, make it more liquid.
- Taste the sauce often during processing or blending. If desired, add more salt or lemon juice.
- Pour the sauce into a bowl once it's blended according to your needed consistency and desired flavor. If desired, stir parley until well mixed or just sprinkle the top with parsley leaves to garnish.

Creamy Fresh Panini

8 Servings

Preparation Time: 16 Minutes

Ingredients:

- 1 jar of 7 oz roasted red peppers, drained and sliced
- 8 slices provolone cheese
- 1 small zucchini, thinly sliced
- 16 slices rustic whole-grain bread
- 4 tbsps finely chopped oil-cured black olives
- ¼ cup chopped fresh basil leaves
- 1 cup Mayonnaise dressing with olive oil, divided

Directions:

- In a small bowl, mix together olives, basil, and mayonnaise dressing.
- Spread the dressing evenly on 4 slices of whole-grain bread.
- Then top it with zucchini, bacon, peppers, and provolone before covering it with another slice of bread.
- Spread the remaining mayonnaise mixture around the bread and cook over medium heat on a nonstick skillet for two minutes on each side or until bread is golden brown on both sides and cheese is melted.

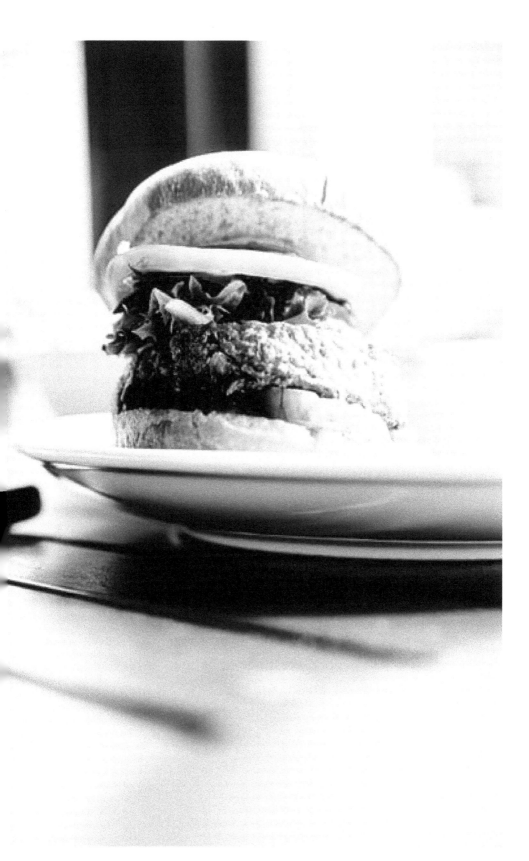

Tuna Panini

2 Servings

Preparation Time: 10 Minutes

Ingredients:

- 1 tbsp softened unsalted butter
- 8 pcs of 1/8-inch kosher dill pickle
- 4 pcs of ¼ inch thick cheddar or Swiss cheese
- Mayonnaise and Dijon mustard
- 2 ciabatta rolls, split
- Pepper and salt
- ½ tsp crushed red pepper
- ½ tbsp minced basil
- ½ tbsp balsamic vinegar
- ¼ cup extra virgin olive oil
- ¼ cup finely diced red onion
- 1 cans of 6oz albacore tuna

Directions:

- Combine the following thoroughly in a bowl: salt pepper, crushed red pepper, basil, vinegar, olive oil, onion, and tuna.
- Smear with mayonnaise and mustard the cut sides of the bread rolls, then layer on: cheese,

tuna salad, and pickles. Cover with the remaining slice of roll.

- Grill in a Panini press, ensuring that cheese is melted and bread is crisped and ridged.

Mangoes with Black Bean Chili

8 Servings

Preparation Time: 10 Minutes

Ingredients:
- 4 tablespoons coconut oil
- 1 onion, chopped
- 4 (25 ounces / 425-g) cans black beans, drained and rinsed
- 2 tablespoons chili powder
- 1 teaspoon sea salt
- ¼ teaspoon freshly ground black pepper
- 1 cup water
- 4 ripe mangoes, sliced thinly
- ¼ cup chopped fresh cilantro, divided
- ¼ cup sliced scallions, divided

Directions:
- Heat the coconut oil in a pot over high heat until melted.
- Put the onion in the pot and sauté for 5 minutes or until translucent.
- Add the black beans to the pot. Sprinkle with chili powder, salt, and ground black pepper. Pour in the water. Stir to mix well.

- Bring to a boil. Reduce the heat to low, then simmering for 5 minutes or until the beans are tender.
- Turn off the heat and mix in the mangoes, then garnish with scallions and cilantro before serving.

Israeli Style Eggplant and Chickpea Salad

12 Servings

Preparation Time: 5 Minutes

Ingredients:

- 4 tablespoons balsamic vinegar
- 4 tablespoons freshly squeezed lemon juice
- 1 teaspoon ground cumin
- ¼ teaspoon sea salt
- 4 tablespoons olive oil, divided
- 1 (1-pound / 454-g) medium globe eggplant, stem removed, cut into flat cubes (about ½ inch thick)
- 1 (15-ounce / 425-g) can chickpeas, drained and rinsed
- ¼ cup chopped mint leaves
- 2 cups sliced sweet onion
- 1 garlic clove, finely minced
- 2 tablespoons sesame seeds, toasted

Directions:

- Preheat the oven to 550ºF (288ºC) or the highest level of your oven or broiler. Grease a baking sheet with 1 tablespoon of olive oil.

- Combine the balsamic vinegar, lemon juice, cumin, salt, and 1 tablespoon of olive oil in a small bowl. Stir to mix well.

- Arrange the eggplant cubes on the baking sheet, then brush with 2 tablespoons of the balsamic vinegar mixture on both sides.

- Broil in the preheated oven for 8 minutes or until lightly browned. Flip the cubes halfway through the cooking time.

- Meanwhile, combine the chickpeas, mint, onion, garlic, and sesame seeds in a large serving bowl. Drizzle with the remaining balsamic vinegar mixture. Stir to mix well.

- Remove the eggplant from the oven. Allow to cool for 5 minutes, then slice them into ½-inch strips on a clean work surface.

- Add the eggplant strips to the serving bowl, then toss to combine well before serving.

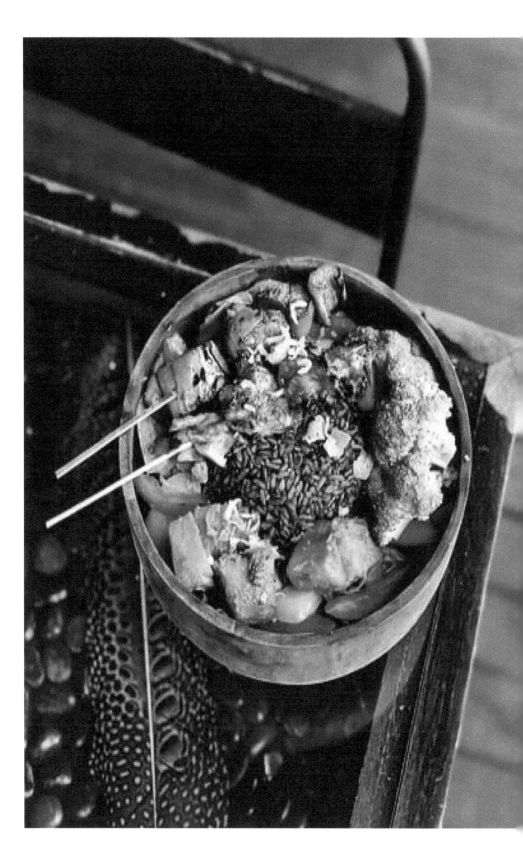

Sautéd Cannellini Beans

12 Servings

Preparation Time: 15 Minutes

Ingredients:

- 4 teaspoons extra-virgin olive oil
- ½ cup minced onion
- ¼ cup red wine vinegar
- 1 (12-ounce / 340-g) can no-salt-added tomato paste
- 4 tablespoons raw honey
- ½ cup of water
- ¼ teaspoon ground cinnamon
- 4 (15-ounce / 425-g) cans cannellini beans

Directions:

- Heat the olive oil in a saucepan over medium heat until shimmering.
- Add the onion and sauté for 5 minutes or until translucent.
- Pour in the red wine vinegar, tomato paste, honey, and water. Sprinkle with cinnamon. Stir to mix well.

- Reduce the heat to low, then pour all the beans into the saucepan. Cook for 10 more minutes. Stir constantly.
- Serve immediately.

Sweet Potato Burgers

8 Servings

Preparation Time: 15 Minutes

Ingredients:

- 2 large sweet potatoes (about 8 ounces/227 g)
- 4 tablespoons extra-virgin olive oil, divided
- 1 cup chopped onion
- 2 large egg
- 1 garlic clove
- 2 cups old-fashioned rolled oats
- 1 tablespoon dried oregano
- 1 tablespoon balsamic vinegar
- ¼ teaspoon kosher salt
- 1 cup crumbled Gorgonzola cheese

Directions:

- Using a fork, pierce the sweet potato all over and microwave on high for 4 to 5 minutes, until softened in the center. Cool slightly before slicing in half.

- Meanwhile, in a large skillet over medium-high heat, heat 1 tablespoon of the olive oil. Add the onion and sauté for 5 minutes.

- Spoon the sweet potato flesh out of the skin and put the flesh in a food processor. Add the cooked onion, egg, garlic, oats, oregano, vinegar, and salt. Pulse until smooth. Add the cheese and pulse four times to barely combine.

- Form the mixture into four burgers. Place the burgers on a plate, and press to flatten each to about ¾-inch thick.

- Wipe out the skillet with a paper towel. Heat the remaining 1 tablespoon of the oil over medium-high heat for about 2 minutes. Add the burgers to the hot oil, then reduce the heat to medium. Cook the burgers for 5 minutes per side.

- Transfer the burgers to a plate and serve.

DINNER

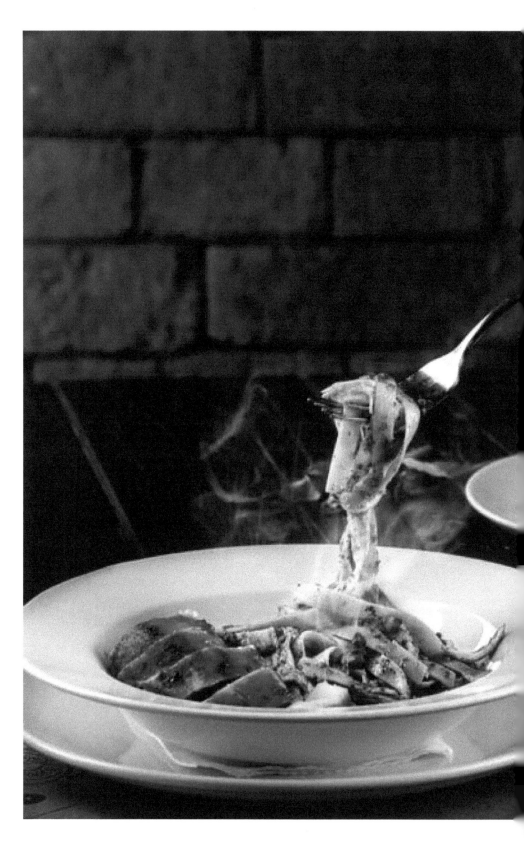

Wild Mushroom Pie Mediterranean

3 Servings

Preparation Time: 20 Minutes

Ingredients:

- 125 grams wild mushrooms, sliced or halved
- 100 grams squash, sliced into small pieces (or pumpkin)
- 1 tablespoon vegetable oil
- 2 tablespoons sundried tomato paste
- 2 small courgettes or zucchini, cut into thin slices
- 8 grams fresh parsley, chopped
- 50 ml cream, dairy-free (I used Oatly)
- 1 large onion, cut in half, and slice finely
- 1 large clove garlic, crushed
- 1 block (500 grams) vegan short-crust pastry (I used JusRol)
- Salt and pepper

Directions:

- Roll out the vegan short-crust pastry and line into a 10-inch baking tray with a loose-bottom. Trim off any excess pastry and then blind bake the pastry at 200C for about 15 minutes. Before filling the tart, remove the baking paper carefully.

- Add vegetable oil into a frying pan. Add the onion and sauté for about 3 to 4 minutes. Put the garlic and the squash; cook for a couple of minutes or until the squash starts to soften. If necessary, add some water. Add the mushrooms, courgettes, and parsley. Carefully stir and season with salt and generously season with pepper.
- Mix the tomato paste with the cream. Stir the mixture into the pan.
- Adjust seasoning according to taste and then transfer into the prepared pastry shell; bake for 20 minutes or until the blind-baked pastry is golden brown.

2 Servings

Preparation Time: 4 Hours

Ingredients:

- 4 whole chicken thighs, including drumstick
- 1 (2-in.) cinnamon stick
- 4 bay leaves
- 16 cups water
- 4 tbsps of salt
- 1 cup extra-virgin olive oil
- 12 cups rehydrated Jew's mallow leaves, drained
- 1 large yellow onion, chopped
- 12 tbs minced garlic
- 1 cup fresh cilantro, finely chopped
- 1 tsp cayenne
- 1 cup fresh lemon juice

Directions:

- In a large pot over medium heat, combine chicken thighs, cinnamon stick, bay leaves, water, and 1 teaspoon salt. Cook for 30 minutes. Skim off any foam that comes to the top.
- Meanwhile, in another large pot over medium heat, heat 1/4 cup extra-virgin

olive oil. Add Jew's mallow leaves, and cook, tossing leaves, for 10 minutes. Remove leaves, and set aside.

- Reduce heat to medium-low. Add remaining 1/4 cup extra-virgin olive oil, yellow onion, and 3 tablespoons garlic, and cook for 5 minutes.
- Return Jew's mallow leaves to onions. Add 8 cups chicken broth strained to the first pot to onions and Jew's mallow leaves in the second pot. Add remaining 1 teaspoon salt, and cook for 1 hour.
- Meanwhile, separate chicken meat from bones. Discard bones and remaining contents of the first pot.
- After leaves have been cooking for 1 hour, add chicken, cilantro, cayenne, and remaining 3 tablespoons garlic, and cook for 20 more minutes.
- Add lemon juice, and cook for 10 more minutes.
- Serve with brown rice.

Fillet O'fish Panini

8 Servings

Preparation Time: 25 Minutes

Ingredients:

- 8 slices thick sourdough bread
- 8 slices mozzarella cheese
- 2 portabella mushroom, sliced
- 1 small onion, sliced
- 12 tbsps oil
- 6 garlic and herb fish fillets

Directions:

- Prepare your fillets by adding salt, pepper, and herbs (rosemary, thyme, parsley, whatever you like), then dredged in flour before deep frying in very hot oil. Once nicely browned, remove from oil and set aside.
- On medium-high fire, sauté for five minutes the onions and mushroom in a skillet with 2 tbsps of oil.
- Prepare sourdough pieces of bread by layering the following over it: cheese, fish

fillet, onion mixture, and cheese again before covering with another bread slice.

- Grill in your Panini press until cheese is melted and bread is crisped and ridged.

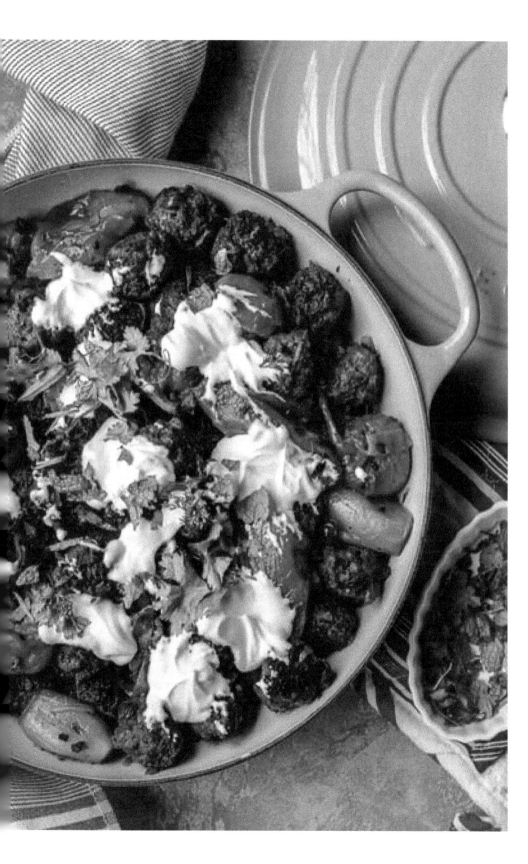

Chicken, Cucumber with Mango Wrap

2 Servings

Preparation Time: 20 Minutes

Ingredients:
- 1 of a medium cucumber cut lengthwise
- 1 of ripe mango
- 2 tbsps salad dressing of choice
- 1 whole wheat tortilla wrap
- 1 inch thick slice of chicken breast around 6 inches in length
- 4 tbsps oil for frying
- 2 tbsps whole wheat flour
- 4 to 4 lettuce leaves
- Salt and pepper to taste

Directions:
- Slice a chicken breast into 1-inch strips and just cook a total of 6-inch strips. That would be like two strips of chicken. Store remaining chicken for future use.
- Season chicken with pepper and salt. Dredge in whole wheat flour.
- On medium fire, place a small and nonstick fry pan and heat oil. Once the oil is hot, add chicken strips and fry until golden brown around 5 minutes per side.

- While the chicken is cooking, place tortilla wraps in the oven and cook for 3 to 5 minutes. Then remove from oven and place on a plate.
- Slice cucumber lengthwise, use only ½ of it and store the remaining cucumber. Peel cucumber cut into quarters and remove the pith. Place the two slices of cucumber on the tortilla wrap, 1-inch away from the edge.
- Slice mango and store the other half with seed. Peel the mango without seed, slice into strips, and place on top of the cucumber on the tortilla wrap.
- Once the chicken is cooked, place the chicken beside the cucumber in a line.
- Add cucumber leaf, drizzle with salad dressing of choice.
- Roll the tortilla wrap, serve and enjoy.

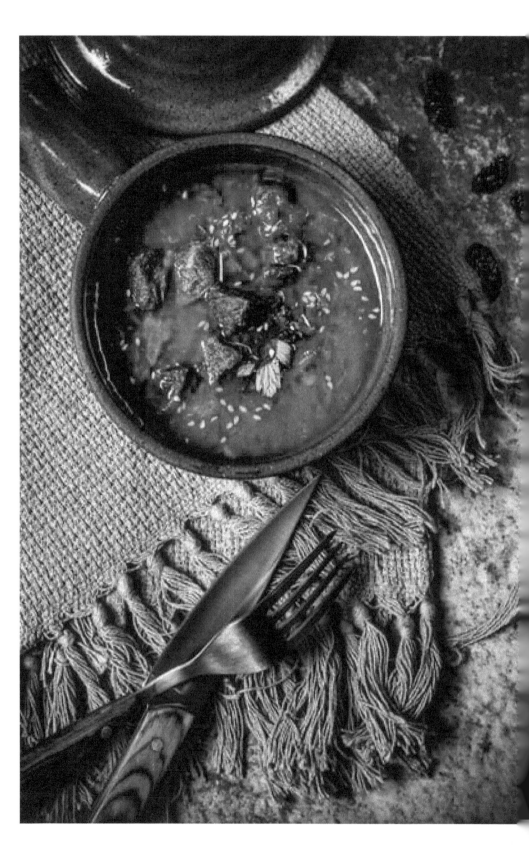

Swordfish Panini with Lemon Aioli

8 Servings

Preparation Time: 25 Minutes

Ingredients:
- 4 oz fresh arugula greens
- 1 loaf focaccia bread
- 2 cloves garlic minced
- 1 tbsp herbes de Provence
- Pepper and salt
- 8 pcs of 6oz swordfish fillet
- 1 ½ tbsps olive oil
- 1 tsp freshly ground black pepper
- ¼ tsp salt
- 1 clove garlic, minced
- 4 tbsps fresh lemon juice
- 1 lemon, zested
- 1 cup mayonnaise

Directions:
- In a small bowl, mix well all lemon Aioli ingredients and put them aside.
- Over medium-high fire, heat olive oil in skillet. Season with pepper, salt, minced garlic, and herbs de Provence the swordfish. Then pan-fry fish until golden brown on both sides, around 5 minutes per side.

- Slice bread into four slices. Smear on the lemon aioli mixture on two bread slices, layer with arugula leaves and fried fish, then cover with the remaining bread slices before grilling in a Panini press.
- Grill until bread is crisped and ridged.

Beans Minestrone

5 Servings

Preparation Time: 1 Hours

Ingredients:

- 1 tablespoon olive oil
- 1 chicken sausages, sliced
- 1 shallot, chopped
- 1 green bell pepper, cored and diced
- 1 garlic clove, chopped
- 1 celery stalks, sliced
- Carrots, diced
- ½ can red beans, drained
- ½ can white beans, drained
- 2 cups chicken stock
- 2 cups water
- 1 cup diced tomatoes
- 1 tablespoon tomato paste
- Salt and pepper to taste
- ½ cup short pasta
- 1 tablespoon lemon juice

Directions:

- Heat the oil in a soup pot and stir in the sausages. Cook for 5 minutes, then add the vegetables.

- Cook for 10 minutes, then add the liquids and season with salt and pepper.
- Cook on low heat for 25 minutes.
- The soup is best served warm or chilled.

Tasty Cauliflower Stew

4 Servings

Preparation Time: 25 Minutes

Ingredients:
- 1 lb ground beef
- 4 tsps salt
- 1 tsp black pepper
- 1 (16-oz.) can plain tomato sauce
- 1 (16-oz.) can crushed tomatoes
- 4 cups water
- 1 tbsp. fresh thyme
- 1 tsp. garlic powder
- 1/2 tsp. onion powder
- 8 cups cauliflower florets
- 2 large potatoes
- 4 large carrots, finely diced
- 1 (16-oz.) can chickpeas, rinsed and drained

Directions:
- In a small bowl, combine beef, 1/2 teaspoon salt, and 1/2 teaspoon black pepper. Form mixture into 20 to 30 mini meatballs about 1 teaspoon each.
- In a large, 3-quart pot over medium heat, add meatballs. Cover and cook for 5 minutes.

- Add tomato sauce, crushed tomatoes, water, thyme, garlic powder, onion powder, remaining 11/2 teaspoons salt, and remaining 1/2 teaspoon black pepper, and simmer for 5 minutes.
- Stir in cauliflower, potatoes, carrots, and chickpeas, and simmer for 20 minutes.
- Serve with brown rice.

Lamb Kebabs Mediterranean

8 Servings

Preparation Time: 40 Minutes

Ingredients:
- 2 pounds ground lamb
- 4 tablespoons scallions, chopped
- 2 tablespoons extra-virgin olive oil
- 2 tablespoons of crème fraîche
- 18 large-sized shallots; peel, halved lengthwise, and then trim root ends but keep intact
- 1/3 cup of water
- 1 teaspoon black pepper, freshly ground
- 2 teaspoons freshly squeezed lemon juice
- 1 tablespoon parsley, flat-leaf, chopped
- 1 garlic clove, minced
- 2 teaspoons salt
- 2 teaspoons pomegranate molasses, divided
- Warm pita bread, for serving

Directions:
- Light an outdoor grill.
- In a medium-sized bowl, gently mix the ground lamb, garlic, crème fraîche, salt, and pepper until combined. With moistened hands, roll lamb mixture to form 16 balls.

- Into 8 pieces 10-inch or less metal skewers, alternate skewer 3 halves shallots and 2 pieces lamb balls. Brush kebabs with olive oil. Place on the grill and cook over medium-high heat for about 3 minutes, turning once, until the outside of the lamb balls and the shallots are browned but are not cooked all the way through.
- Transfer the semi-cooked kebabs into a very large-sized deep skillet, about 12-14 inches. Add water, lemon juice, and 1 teaspoon pomegranate molasses to the water; bring the water mixture to a boil. When boiling, cover and gently simmer for about 30 minutes over low flame or heat or until the meatballs are cooked through, and the shallots are very tender.
- Uncover the skillet; increase heat to high. Add remaining 1/2 teaspoon pomegranate molasses. Continue cooking for 5 minutes more, basting the shallots and the meatballs occasionally until they are glazed.
- Transfer kebabs into a serving platter. Drizzle with the remaining sauce from the skillet. Garnish with parsley and scallions. Serve with warmed pita bread.

DESSERT

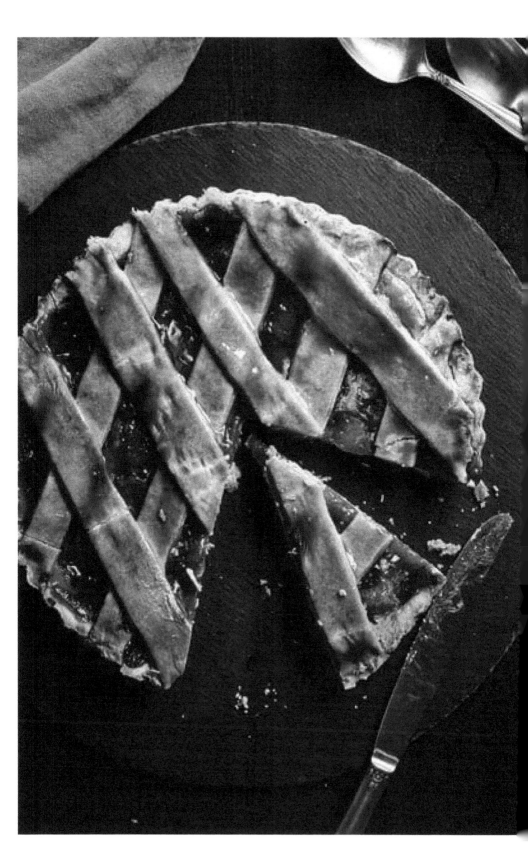

Cranberry, Banana, and Oat Bars

16 Servings

Preparation Time: 15 Minutes

Ingredients:

- 5 tablespoons, 4 extra-virgin olive oil
- 5 medium ripe bananas, mashed
- 1 cup almond butter
- 1 cup maple syrup
- 1 cup dried cranberries
- 2 cups old-fashioned rolled oats
- ¼ cup oat flour
- ¼ cup ground flaxseed
- ¼ teaspoon ground cloves
- 1 cup shredded coconut
- 1 teaspoon ground cinnamon
- 1 teaspoon vanilla extract

Directions:

- Preheat the oven to 400ºF (205ºC). Line a 8-inch square pan with parchment paper, then grease with olive oil.
- Combine the mashed bananas, almond butter, and maple syrup in a bowl. Stir to mix well.
- Mix in the remaining ingredients and stir to mix well until thick and sticky.

- Spread the mixture evenly on the square pan with a spatula, then bake in the preheated oven for 40 minutes or until a toothpick inserted in the center comes out clean.
- Remove them from the oven and slice them into 16 bars to serve.

Berry with Rhubarb Cobbler

16 Servings

Preparation Time: 25 Minutes

Ingredients:

- 2 cups fresh raspberries
- 4 cups fresh blueberries
- 1 cup sliced (½-inch) rhubarb pieces
- 1 tablespoon arrowroot powder
- ¼ cup unsweetened apple juice
- 4 tablespoons melted coconut oil
- ¼ cup raw honey
- 2 cups almond flour
- 2 tablespoons arrowroot powder
- 1 cup shredded coconut
- ¼ cup raw honey
- 1 cup coconut oil

Directions:

- Make the Cobbler
- Preheat the oven to 350ºF (180ºC). Grease a baking dish with melted coconut oil.
- Combine the ingredients for the cobbler in a large bowl. Stir to mix well.
- Spread the mixture in a single layer on the baking dish. Set aside.

- Make the Topping
- Combine the almond flour, arrowroot powder, and coconut in a bowl. Stir to mix well.
- Fold in the honey and coconut oil. Stir with a fork until the mixture crumbled.
- Spread the topping over the cobbler, then bake in the preheated oven for 35 minutes or until frothy and golden brown.
- Serve immediately.

Citrus Cranberry and Quinoa Energy Bites

3 Serving

Preparation Time: 25 Minutes

Ingredients:

- 1 tablespoon almond butter
- 1 tablespoon maple syrup
- ¾ cup cooked quinoa
- ½ tablespoon dried cranberries
- ½ tablespoon chia seeds
- ¼ cup ground almonds
- ¼ cup sesame seeds, toasted
- Zest of 1 orange
- ½ teaspoon vanilla extract

Directions:

- Line a baking sheet with parchment paper.
- Combine the butter and maple syrup in a bowl. Stir to mix well.
- Fold in the remaining ingredients and stir until the mixture holds together and smooth.
- Divide the mixture into 12 equal parts, then shape each part into a ball.
- Arrange the balls on the baking sheet, then refrigerate for at least 15 minutes.
- Serve chilled.

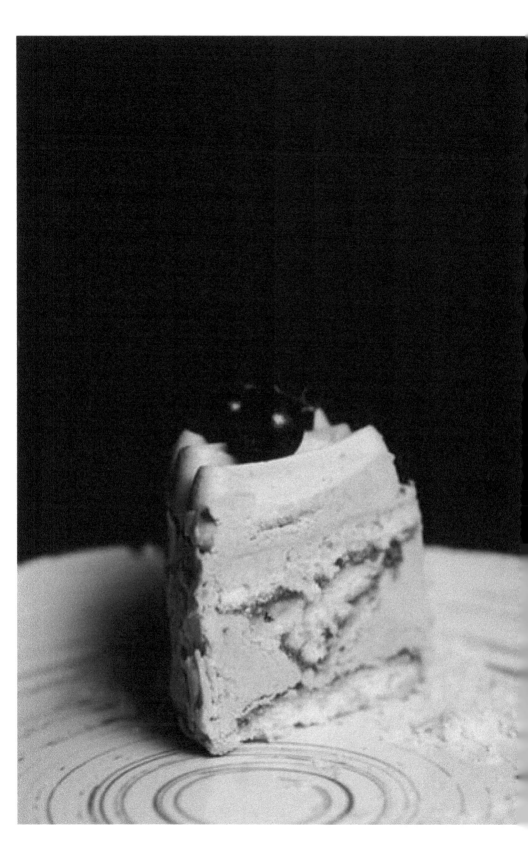

Avocado and Chocolate Mousse

10 Servings

Preparation Time: 40 Minutes

Ingredients:

- 16 ounces (227 g) dark chocolate (60% cocoa or higher), chopped
- ¼ cup unsweetened coconut milk
- 4 tablespoons coconut oil
- 4 ripe avocados, deseeded
- ¼ cup raw honey
- Sea salt, to taste

Directions:

- Put the chocolate in a saucepan. Pour in the coconut milk and add the coconut oil.
- Cook for 3 minutes or until the chocolate and coconut oil melt. Stir constantly.
- Put the avocado in a food processor, then drizzle with honey and melted chocolate. Pulse to combine until smooth.
- Pour the mixture into a serving bowl, then sprinkle with salt. Refrigerate to chill for 30 minutes and serve.

Oat Crisp and Blueberry

8 Servings

Preparation Time: 15 Minutes

Ingredients:

- 8 tablespoons coconut oil, melted, plus more for greasing
- 8 cups fresh blueberries
- Juice of ½ lemon
- 4 teaspoons lemon zest
- ¼ cup maple syrup
- 1 cup gluten-free rolled oats
- 1 cup chopped pecans
- 1 teaspoon ground cinnamon
- Sea salt, to taste

Directions:

- Preheat the oven to 350ºF (180ºC). Grease a baking sheet with coconut oil.
- Combine the blueberries, lemon juice and zest, and maple syrup in a bowl. Stir to mix well, then spread the mixture on the baking sheet.

- Combine the remaining ingredients in a small bowl. Stir to mix well. Pour the mixture over the blueberries mixture.
- Bake in the preheated oven for 20 minutes or until the oats are golden brown.
- Serve immediately with spoons.

Hazelnuts with Glazed Pears

8 Servings

Preparation Time: 10 Minutes

Ingredients:

- 8 pears, peeled, cored, and quartered lengthwise
- 2 cups apple juice
- 2 tablespoons grated fresh ginger
- 1 cup pure maple syrup
- ¼ cup chopped hazelnuts

Directions:

- Put the pears in a pot, then pour in the apple juice. Bring to a boil over medium-high heat, then reduce the heat to medium-low. Stir constantly.
- Cover and simmer for an additional 15 minutes or until the pears are tender.
- Meanwhile, combine the ginger and maple syrup in a saucepan. Bring to a boil over medium-high heat. Stir frequently. Turn off the heat and transfer the syrup to a small bowl and let sit until ready to use.

- Transfer the pears into a large serving bowl with a slotted spoon, then top the pears with syrup.
- Spread the hazelnuts over the pears and serve immediately.

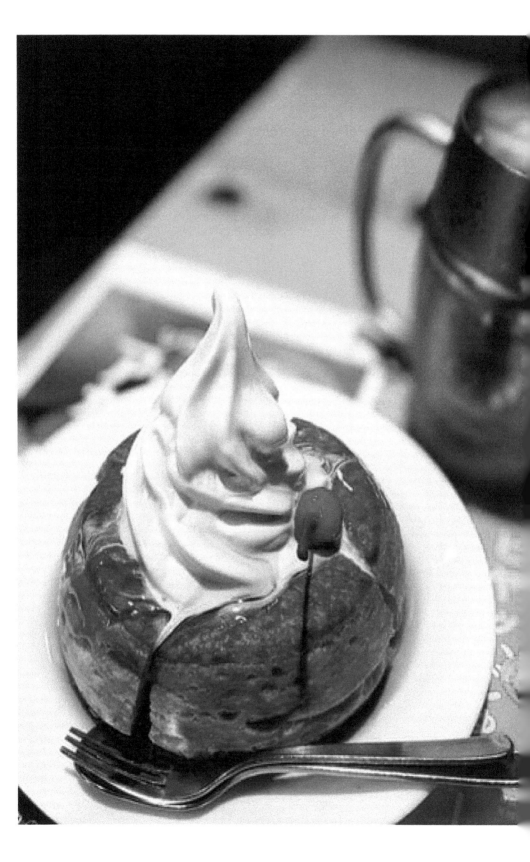

Blackberry Lemony Granita

4 Servings

Preparation Time: 10 Minutes

Ingredients:

- 2 pounds (454 g) fresh blackberries
- 1 teaspoon chopped fresh thyme
- ¼ cup freshly squeezed lemon juice
- 1 cup raw honey
- 1 cup water

Directions:

- Put all the ingredients in a food processor, then pulse to purée.
- Pour the mixture through a sieve into a baking dish. Discard the seeds that remain in the sieve.
- Put the baking dish in the freezer for 2 hours. Remove the dish from the refrigerator and stir to break any frozen parts.
- Return the dish back to the freezer for an hour, then stir to break any frozen parts again.
- Return the dish to the freezer for 4 hours until the granita is completely frozen.
- Remove it from the freezer and mash to serve.

Biscotti Mediterranean

6 Servings

Preparation Time: 60 Minutes

Ingredients:

- 4 eggs
- 1 cup whole-wheat flour
- 1 cup all-purpose flour
- Three-quarters cup parmesan cheese, grated.
- 4 tsps. baking powder
- 2 tbsps. sugar
- ¼ cup sun-dried tomato finely chopped.
- ¼ cup Kalamata olive finely chopped.
- 1 cup olive oil
- Half tsp of.salt.
- Half tsp of black pepper, cracked.
- 1 tsp dried oregano (preferably Greek)
- 2 tsps dried basil

Directions:

- Into a large-sized bowl, beat the eggs and the sugar together.
- Transfer in the olive; beat until smooth.
- In another bowl, combine the flours, baking powder, pepper, salt, oregano, and basil.

- Mix the flour mix into the egg mixture, mixing until Keep blending ed.
- Mix in the cheese, tomatoes, and olives; mixing until thoroughly combined.
- Divide the dough into 2 portions: shape each into 10-inch-long logs.
- Place the logs into a parchment-lined cookie sheet; flatten the log tops slightly.
- Bake for about 30 minutes in a preheated 375F oven or until the logs are pale golden and not quite firm to the touch.
- Remove from the oven; let cool on the baking sheet for 3 minutes.
- Transfer the logs into a cutting board; slice each log into Half-inch diagonal slices using a serrated knife.
- Place the biscotti slices on the baking sheet, return into the 325F oven, and bake for about 20 to 25 minutes until dry and firm.
- Flip the slices halfway through baking.
- Remove from the oven, transfer on a wire rack, and let cool.

Orange Cardamom Cookies

16 Servings

Preparation Time: 12 minutes

Ingredients:
- 1cup whole-wheat flour
- 1 cup all-purpose flour
- 2 large eggs
- 1 tablespoon sesame seeds, toasted, optional (salted roasted pistachios, chopped)
- 1 tsp. orange zest
- 1 tsp. vanilla extract
- 1 cup butter, softened.
- 1 cup of sugar.
- ¼ tsp. ground cardamom

Directions:

- Preheat the oven to 375F.
- In a medium bowl, Keep blending the orange zest and the sugar thoroughly, and then Keep blending in the cardamom.
- Add the butter and with a mixer, beat until the mixture is fluffy and light.
- Beat in the egg and the vanilla into the mixture.
- With the mixer on low speed, mix the flour into the mixture.

- Line 3 baking sheets with parchment paper. Using a level tsp measure, drop batter of the cookie mixture onto the sheets.
- Top each cookie with a pinch of sesame seeds or nuts, if desired; bake for about 10-12 minutes or until the cookies are brown at the edges and crisp.
- When baked, transfer the cookies to a cooling rack and let them cool completely.

SALADS AND SOUPS

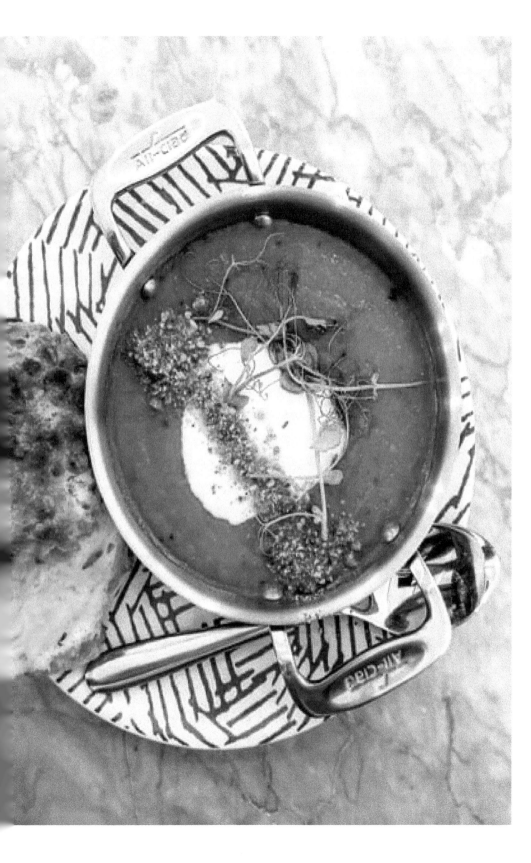

Cheesy Zucchini Soup

4 Servings

Preparation Time: 20 Minutes

Ingredients:

- 1 medium onion, peeled and chopped
- 2 cups bone broth
- 1 tablespoon coconut oil
- 2 zucchinis, cut into chunks
- 1 tablespoon nutritional yeast
- Dash of black pepper
- 1 tablespoon parsley, chopped, for garnish
- 1 tablespoon coconut cream, for garnish

Directions:

- Melt the coconut oil in a large pan over medium heat and add onions.
- Sauté for about 3 minutes and add zucchinis and bone broth.
- Reduce the heat to simmer for about 15 minutes and cover the pan.
- Add the nutritional yeast and transfer it to an immersion blender.
- Blend until smooth and season with black pepper.
- Top with coconut cream and parsley to serve.

Peppers Salad

12 Servings

Preparation Time: 10 Minutes

Ingredients:

- 4 green bell peppers, cut into thick strips
- 4 red bell peppers, cut into thick strips
- 2 tablespoons olive oil
- 2 garlic cloves, minced
- 1 cup goat cheese, crumbled
- A pinch of salt and black pepper

Directions:

- In a bowl, mix the bell peppers with the garlic and the other ingredients, toss and serve.

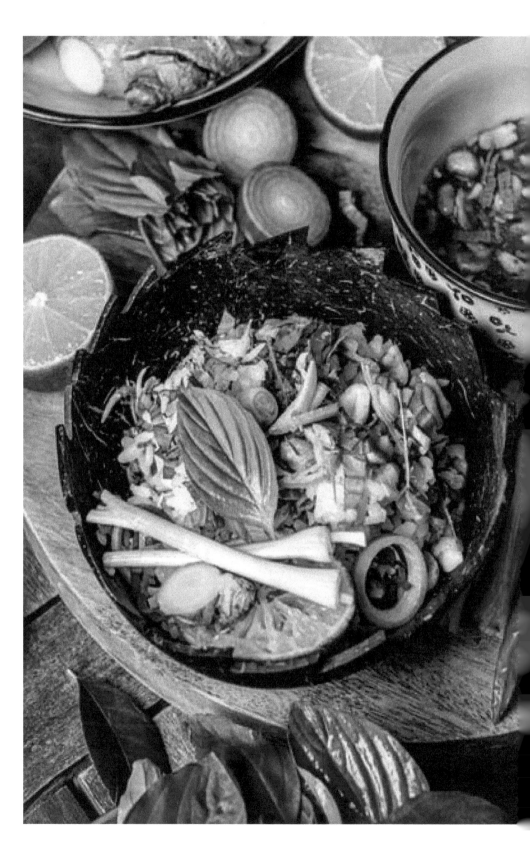

Arugula & Salmon Salad

4 Servings

Preparation Time: 12 Minutes

Ingredients:

- ¼ cup red onion, sliced thinly
- 2 tbsps fresh lemon juice
- 1 ½ tbsps olive oil
- 2 tbsps extra-virgin olive oil
- 1 tbsp red wine vinegar
- 2 center-cut salmon fillets (6-oz each)
- 1 cup cherry tomato, halved
- 6 cups baby arugula leaves
- Pepper and salt to taste

Directions:

- In a shallow bowl, mix pepper, salt, 1 ½ tbsps olive oil, and lemon juice. Toss in salmon fillets and rub with the marinade. Allow to marinate for at least 15 minutes.
- Grease a baking sheet and preheat the oven to 350°F.

- Bake marinated salmon fillet for 10 to 12 minutes or until flaky with skin side touching the baking sheet.
- Meanwhile, in a salad bowl, mix onion, tomatoes, and arugula.
- Season with pepper and salt. Drizzle with vinegar and oil. Toss to combine and serve right away with baked salmon on the side.

BBQ Chicken Pizza Soup

12 Servings

Preparation Time: 1 Hour and 30 Minutes

Ingredients:
- 12 chicken legs
- 1 medium red onion, diced
- 8 garlic cloves
- 1 large tomato, unsweetened
- 8 cups green beans
- ¾ cup BBQ Sauce
- 1½ cups mozzarella cheese, shredded
- 1 cup ghee
- 4 quarts water
- 4 quarts chicken stock
- Salt and black pepper, to taste
- Fresh cilantro, for garnishing

Directions:
- Put chicken, water, and salt in a large pot and bring to a boil.
- Reduce the heat to medium-low and cook for about 75 minutes.
- Shred the meat off the bones using a fork and keep aside.
- Put ghee, red onions, and garlic in a large soup and cook over a medium heat.

- Add chicken stock and bring to a boil over high heat.
- Add green beans and tomato to the pot and cook for about 15 minutes.
- Add BBQ Sauce, shredded chicken, salt, and black pepper to the pot.
- Ladle the soup into serving bowls and top with shredded mozzarella cheese and cilantro to serve.

Garden Mediterranean Salad

4 Servings

Preparation Time: 5 Minutes

Ingredients:

- 12 cups mixed greens
- 4 cups cherry tomatoes, halved
- 1 medium red onion, sliced (1/2 cup)
- 3 tbsps tahini paste
- 6 tbsps fresh lemon juice
- 3 tbsps balsamic vinegar
- 6 tbsps plus 1 tsp. extra-virgin olive oil
- 6 tbsps of water
- 1 tsp. salt
- 1 tsp fresh ground black pepper
- 1 cup pine nuts

Directions:

- In a large bowl, add mixed greens, cherry tomatoes, and red onion.
- In a small bowl, whisk together tahini paste, lemon juice, balsamic vinegar, 3 tablespoons extra-virgin olive oil, water, salt, and black pepper.
- Preheat a small skillet over medium-low heat for 1 minute. Add remaining 1 teaspoon extra-virgin olive oil and pine

nuts, and cook, stirring to toast evenly on all sides, for 4 minutes. Transfer pine nuts to a plate, and let cool for 2 minutes.

- Pour dressing over vegetables, and toss to coat evenly. Top with toasted pine nuts, and serve immediately.

Olives Squash Soup

5 Servings

Preparation Time: 45 Minutes

Ingredients:

- 1½ cups beef bone broth
- 1 small onion, peeled and grated.
- ½ teaspoon sea salt
- ¼ teaspoon poultry seasoning
- 2 small Delicata Squash, chopped
- 2 garlic cloves, minced
- 2 tablespoons olive oil
- ¼ teaspoon black pepper
- 1 small lemon, juiced
- 5 tablespoons sour cream

Directions:

- Put Delicata Squash and water in a medium pan and bring to a boil.
- Reduce the heat and cook for about 20 minutes.
- Drain and set aside.
- Put olive oil, onions, garlic, and poultry seasoning in a small saucepan.
- Cook for about 2 minutes and add broth.
- Allow it to simmer for 5 minutes and remove from heat.

- Whisk in the lemon juice and transfer the mixture into a blender.
- Pulse until smooth and top with sour cream.

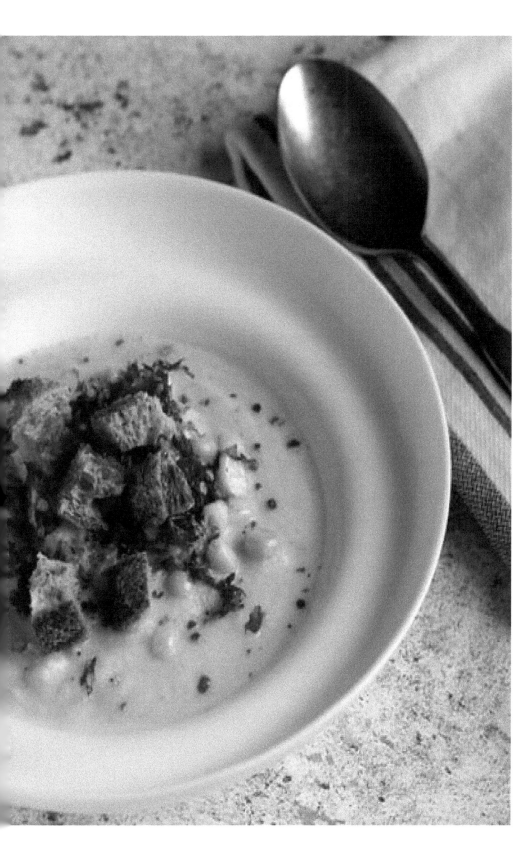

Spicy Tomato Halibut Soup

16 Servings

Preparation Time: 1 Hour and 5 Minutes

Ingredients:

- 4 garlic cloves, minced
- 2 tablespoons of olive oil
- ¼ cup fresh parsley, chopped
- 10 anchovies canned in oil, minced
- 12 cups vegetable broth
- 1 teaspoon of black pepper
- 1poundhalibut fillets, chopped
- 6 tomatoes, peeled and diced
- 1 teaspoon of salt
- 1 teaspoon of red chili flakes

Directions:

- Heat olive oil in a large stockpot over medium heat and add garlic and half of the parsley.
- Add anchovies, tomatoes, vegetable broth, red chili flakes, salt, and black pepper, and bring to a boil.
- Reduce the heat to medium-low and simmer for about 20 minutes.
- Add halibut fillets and cook for about 10 minutes.

- Dish out the halibut and shred it into small pieces.
- Mix back with the soup and garnish with the remaining fresh parsley to serve.

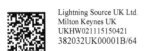
Lightning Source UK Ltd.
Milton Keynes UK
UKHW021115150421
382032UK00001B/64

9 781802 525076